ALKALIN]

Original Alkaline J____, _____ies,

and Teas

Rebalance your pH in 7 Days or Less

THE ALKALINE DIET LIFESTYLE

SERIES BOOK 5

By Marta Tuchowska

Copyright ©Marta Tuchowska 2015

www.holisticwellnessproject.com

www.alkalinedietlifestyle.com

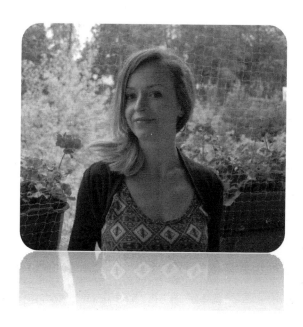

TABLE OF CONTENTS

Your Free Complimentary Alkaline Diet Guide + Vegan Alkaline Recipes+ Charts

Revolutionize Your Life with Alkaline Foods!

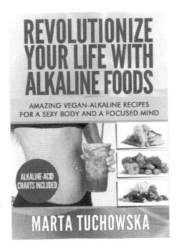

This eBook Will Help You Transform Your Body, Restore Energy and Take Your Health to a Whole New Level!

Grab your free copy today from:
http://bit.ly/AlkalineMarta

INTRODUCTION

Dear Reader,

Thank you for taking an interest in my book!

The purpose of this book is to share with you just how easy it is to keep yourself nicely energized with the aid of alkaline drinks, smoothies and juices. There is no need to drink gallons of coffee or energy drinks. These only make your body more acidic, therefore even more tired and prone to all kinds of illnesses.

One of the biggest challenges that people of the 21st century are facing is low energy levels. This comes as an unpleasant package - one negative condition or reaction leads to another, into a cycle of negativity and unhealthiness in the mind and body. This can include weight gain, lack of focus, irritability, headaches, insomnia, and more.

I am a holistic wellness coach fascinated with the Alkaline Diet and inspire personal transformations through a holistic lifestyle. Originally, I worked as a certified massage therapist.

Many of my clients would ask me about diets and what they can specifically eat to feel more energized on a daily basis.

A healthy lifestyle will lead to a happier and better life. Even if you have a lucrative career, but you find it hard to crawl out of bed every morning, how can you enjoy your life? If you have little energy and feel unhealthy, you will not feel as motivated to socialize and start new relationships. Pursuing new careers or travels, and running a business seems like something impossible. Health is wealth and wealth is health.

Start right here and right now. Think as an investor, not a consumer. On a daily basis, you will need to make simple, healthy choices. As an investor, you select what suits you and your overall health, and you will reap the rewards for years to come. This is a general health and wellness message that I try to convey through all my books, courses, and programs as well as through my blog located at holisticwellnessproject.com. If you are interested in body and mind transformation I strongly recommend you check out the blog for inspiration, motivation and information.

Wellness and health is about understanding, practicing and sharing your personal experiences with other people, and following through with your decisions. This is what I am trying to do. Many people might be skeptical of my alkaline diet and think that it comes naturally for me. In reality, I very much enjoy my alkaline diet but I still have temptations that are not part of the diet. I stay motivated and strong to follow through with my diet because I have had lasting energy and healthfulness - there are also mental and emotional benefits, something I talk about in my course AlkalineDietLifestyle.com

This is a never-ending journey but I am committed to it, and since you are reading this book, I am 100% sure that you will be committed to it as well.

I have an example that you can probably relate to - this morning was pretty rainy and cold. My first temptation was to crawl out of bed and to indulge in coffee or super strong black tea. There was an internal struggle in my mind! Instead, I CHOSE to take my energy levels into consideration. Truthfully, I felt a bit tired, and my week has been hectic. I have been working really long hours on my projects, and working out every day. I had to take care of the house (my partner broke his hand) and I was also helping a friend move houses. To add even more to the chaos I was also coaching clients. What a busy agenda!

Here's how I worked through this conundrum. I knew that if I went for this cup of coffee (which is in my house only because my boyfriend enjoys a cup or two every now and then), I would get an energy crash after a few hours and feel even more tired in the afternoon. As a result, I'd probably skip the gym. You see, these things have happened in the past, so I was familiar with what the results would be. Despite this struggle, I took my own advice. I first hydrated myself with a few glasses of alkaline water (I use special filters that alkalize water- the best health investment I have ever made) with lemon juice, then I stretched my body, breathed and finally decided on a massive alkaline green smoothie followed by a healthy, balanced breakfast (I don't live entirely on smoothies and I don't recommend you do). I felt like my optimal pH levels were back. I was focused, working, and happy. I call this being "fully on track" and enjoying it.

There are going to be plenty of battles when your emotions will be telling you to do something you know is not healthy, and you will probably succumb to those temptations more than a few times. Just remember, failure also leads to success. It's up to you if you want to use the results of your battles – both wins and losses - as an asset and learn something from them.

If you are healthy and balanced, you can still enjoy an occasional glass of wine or a cup of coffee or tea (make sure it's organic, fair trade). Should you choose a cup of coffee, add some almond milk to keep it more alkaline, as coffee is acidic. However, this should be a treat that you choose, not a habit... You are in control of your health; don't let unhealthy choices control you.

In my experience, the healthier and more alkaline you go, the less temptations you will experience. A body that is well-fed and has a healthy, balanced pH level that does not lack nutrients feels at peace. Thus, it does not bother you when your mind screams, "I am hungry! Get a take away kebab or pizza!," or, "I need more energy. Get me a big creamy coffee." If your body is not balanced, it lacks energy and nutrients. This leads to cravings for more sugar, caffeine, processed foods, you name it! If you keep your pH balanced, you will not have as many of these craving and you will be able to say, "no" to those poor choices.

This book is designed as an Alkaline Wellness Guide for those who are interested in:

- the alkaline diet
- naturopathy
- commencing the journey towards a healthy lifestyle
- wellness and fitness
- increasing their energy levels to restore balance and zest for life

I would also invite those who are following:

- A gluten free diet
- A vegan diet
- The Paleo diet.

The teachings in this book will be compatible with your nutritional choices and patterns (including dairy free and gluten free).

I understand that there are many nutritional ways and beliefs, but the most important thing is to <u>find what works for you</u>. I found my wellness success in the Alkaline Diet. I feel so passionate about sharing my recipes, tips and personal experiences to help you create a healthier version of yourself with the Alkaline Diet.

Take what you like from this book and reject the rest. I am not telling you what to do - I am telling you what I do.

My belief is that everyone can benefit from adding more alkaline foods and drinks to their everyday routine. This is something that can be combined with your other diets and nutritional patterns.

"There is only one disease - the constant over-acidification of the body." – Dr. Robert O. Young

IMPORTANT:

- This is not a diet plan or a detailed detox program. I believe that these need to be designed specifically for each person.
- The alkaline ingredients in this book heal you from the inside out.
- The balanced Alkaline Diet uses the "80/20 Rule". It means that you should stick to 80% of alkaline foods and 20% acidic foods (the food must be unprocessed). If you are already healthy and balanced, you can occasionally make it 70% alkaline and 30% acidic.
- Alkaline smoothies made of organic alkaline fruit (less sugar, 100% alkaline) and vegetables are the best and the fastest way to get on a healthy track and as a result you can also lose weight naturally. It's all about balancing your pH level. There is no calorie counting on the Alkaline Diet (thankfully!) and supplements are optional.
- The Alkaline Diet has recently gotten popular thanks to the "new biology" research of Doctor Robert O. Young (I highly recommend you check out his books). Additionally, celebrities and actors including Victoria Beckham and celebrity public speakers like Tony

Robbins follow the Alkaline Diet. However, it has been around for decades!

Naturopathy is very popular in Spain, especially in Barcelona where I am based. There are plenty of schools, naturopathy centers and famous naturopathic doctors. It's thanks to living here that I decided to study natural therapies (thanks Spain!). My research led me back to the 70s, where many local alternative health practitioners recommended alkaline water and other alkaline drinks including smoothies made of veggies and non-acidic fruits to treat various conditions of the digestive track as well as skin problems, impotence and even anxiety. I have read and researched in Polish and German and again I bumped into the same naturopathic formulas, using the ingredients that we will be using in this book. They did not always call it the Alkaline Diet back then, but they knew that certain foods can increase or decrease our energy levels..

I am very open and direct in telling people about my experiences; I know that people relate better to real world situations. You can contact me anytime. The back end if this book contains my contact info (even my personal Facebook page - I am 100% transparent so that you know I am a real human being facing the same challenges as you may be). So, don't be a stranger, come and say. "Hi!" I encourage you to start taking notes now and contact me later, after reading this book. It's like a free consultation for my readers and I am here to lend you a hand.

My objective is not only to provide you with information but also with inspiration and motivation. The first challenge for you is to learn which foods are alkaline. My tips will help you create your own natural alkaline energizers.

I suppose that you are reading this book as you have been neglecting your diet for a long time and your body really needs huge amounts of alkalinity. Maybe you spent the last weekend partying at your best friend's wedding and your body still feels a bit "not there". Maybe you went on vacation and indulged in foods that were unhealthy. Maybe you were visiting family or friends who have a more "traditional" (meat and potatoes) view of nutrition and you stuffed yourself with all kinds of meats, plenty of desserts and possibly processed foods. Maybe you had a really stressful week at work, and now it's your weekend or time off and you want to create your holistic wellness spa at home (I have a series of books specifically to teach you how to do it inexpensively in order to rejuvenate your body and mind) and want to heal from the inside out with a myriad of alkaline smoothies? No matter which category you belong to, I welcome you all. This is going to be a really exciting journey.

****
****

The alkaline diet is based on the basic principle that, if the pH level in your body is unbalanced, it can cause many health problems, ranging from weight gain and no energy, to headaches and arthritis. Your pH level can range from zero, which is completely acidic, to 14, completely alkaline. Ideally, your pH level should be neutral at 7, but healthy blood should have a pH level around 7.35. When your pH level falls below 7, it can cause symptoms, such as low energy, **anxiety,** and aches and pains in your body. The main factor affecting your pH level is your diet, since the foods you eat can make your pH level more acidic. The alkaline diet seeks to correct this, by increasing your consumption of alkalinizing foods. Ideally, some 75% to 80% of your diet should consist of alkaline foods, while the remaining 20% to 25% can be acidic.

You can check your pH level by using pH test strips at your local drugstore. These strips are made with litmus paper, which change color when dipped into your urine, showing how acidic or alkaline your pH level is. When it changes color, compare it with the color chart on the box to find the reading. Generally, you should test your pH level once a day. Do it first thing in the morning, before you have eaten anything. Write down the results in a journal or chart, so that you can determine how the alkaline diet is affecting your pH level. If you find your pH levels to be highly abnormal, however, you should consult with your doctor, as this may be a sign of a more serious health problem.

Once you have gotten used to the alkaline diet, you won't even need to check your pH using urine strips. You will know it by the way you feel and your energy and focus. Your body will then crave more alkaline foods naturally. It took me only a few months to transition to this state, which, I must admit, is great. My body is demanding healthy foods all the time.

If this is your first exposure to the Alkaline Diet (I understand that it can be complicated to begin this journey), I suggest you check out these blog posts I have written for beginners:

http://www.holisticwellnessproject.com/blog/alkaline-diet-2/

or visit: www.holisticwellnessproject.com click on "blog" and select a category you are interested in:

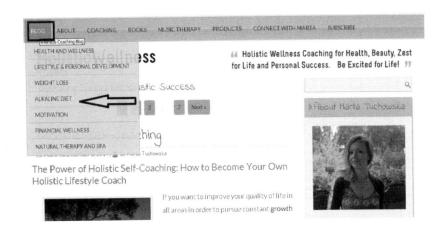

I especially recommend you get basic alkaline charts from my blog post:

http://www.holisticwellnessproject.com/blog/alkaline-diet-2/alkaline-foods-wellness/

Print them out and stick them on your refrigerator.

You can also check out the rest of my books from "The Alkaline Diet Lifestyle" series. This is book number 5, the rest being:

- How to Lose Massive Weight with the Alkaline Diet
- The Alkaline Satisfaction Cookbook
- Alkaline Diet Motivation

- The Alkaline Diet Spiced Up! (Alkaline-Asian Recipes)

(You will find them at:
www.amazom.com/author/mtuchowska)

The above mentioned resources are optional supplements. For now, focus on energizing with the alkaline foods discussed in this book. Our number one goal is to make you energized and bouncing off the walls. This is totally possible. You can even re-balance your pH level in 7 days or less. Of course, if you suffer from any serious diseases or have been eating unhealthy it may take longer to get your optimal pH level back, but you will feel more energetic only after a few days.

"Good Health" is an asset that can never be taken for granted as you never know when you might run out of it. To prevent such a situation from coming about, make sure you "alkalize" as much as possible. Your diet should consist of at least 70% alkaline foods, 80% alkaline being optimal. In order to help you gain control over your body, you must cut out all processed acidic foods from your diet (add to it caffeine, sodas and artificial energy drinks) since an acidic environment inside the body is extremely ideal for a whole array of diseases.

Therefore, to help prevent the onset of these conditions, you must cleanse your body and increase the level of alkaline. Eating foods that fall under the category of alkaline is your best bet to fight away all of the acid. The acidic foods can wreak havoc in your body and end up corroding it from the inside out.

Balancing yourself with alkaline drinks, is the quickest way to get your energy back. Do a one week challenge - eliminate caffeine, sodas and sugary drinks. Add at least one alkaline juice and alkaline smoothie a day. Remember to drink plenty of water and eat wholesome, unprocessed foods. It's really easy and soon you will be bouncing off the walls. Energy is something that we all need to create successful lifestyles, right?

Once you look at the chart, which separates the acidic from the alkaline, you will be surprised to see just how many of the acidic substances you consume on a daily basis.

In this book we look at over 45 creative recipes of healing alkaline drinks, which are meant to remove toxins, cleanse your body and help you achieve your wellness and weight loss goals faster.

If you are on medication, suffer from any serious condition, have undergone surgery or are just about to undergo one, are new to dieting, especially the alkaline diet, are pregnant/lactating, consult a physician first.

Let's dive into it! Make sure you start practicing as soon as you can!

ALKALINE SHOPPING LIST

Here's your shopping list. Opt for fresh and organic fruits and vegetables. Ordering items online may save time, or you may visit your local farmers' market. You can also order more and split with your neighbors and family to cut down costs. When it comes to fruits and vegetables, the fresher they are the better. I usually buy new fruits and vegetables every 2-3 days max. If you can grow your own (something that I am learning now), that's even better and 100% organic and fresh.

ALKALINE INGREDIENTS

"Super Quick Shopping List for Modern People"

These ingredients are super alkaline. I suggest you make them your priority.

Here's the list of HIGH alkaline foods:

Alkaline Veggies:

- Beetroot
- Capsicum/Pepper
- Cabbage
- Celery
- Chives

- Collard/Spring Greens
- Endive
- Garlic
- Ginger
- Lettuce
- Mustard Greens
- Okra
- Onion
- Radish
- Red Onion
- Rocket/Arugula
- Wakame seaweed
- Spinach and Kale
- Artichokes (although hard to use them in smoothies, it can be done)
- Asparagus
- Carrot
- Courgette/Zucchini
- Leeks
- Pumpkin
- Rutabaga
- Squash
- Watercress

These are NEUTRAL alkaline foods and can also be used in your smoothies:

- Cantaloupe
- Fresh Dates
- Nectarine
- Plum
- Sweet Cherry (Black Cherry)
- Watermelon
- Millet (not for Paleo people)
- Oats/Oatmeal (not for Paleo people)
- Spelt grain(not for Paleo people)
- Brown Rice (not for Paleo people)
- Rice & Soy Milk (not for Paleo people)
- Brazil Nuts
- Pecan Nuts
- Hazel Nuts
- Grapeseed Oil

SMOOTHIE INGREDIENTS:

Alkaline Fruits:
- Avocado
- Tomato
- Lemon
- Lime

- Grapefruit
- Fresh Coconut
- Pomegranate

Other Alkaline Smoothie Ingredients you might need:

- Herbal teas (cooled down)
- Herbs (basil, coriander, curry, rosemary, mint, thyme...)
- Almond milk
- Goat milk (if you can digest it, but I suggest you choose vegan options)
- Coconut water
- Coconut milk

OILS:

Don't forget about oils- these are "good oils":

- Avocado Oil
- Coconut Oil
- Flax Oil
- Udo's Oil
- Olive Oil

Alkaline nuts and seeds for more nutrients in your smoothies:

- Almonds
- Coconut
- Flax Seeds
- Pumpkin Seeds
- Sesame Seeds
- Sunflower Seeds

Alkaline smoothies are also great with some:

- Quinoa
- Millet
- Amaranth

However, these ingredients are not compatible with Paleo Diet inspired lifestyles.

If you are pressed for time, resort to these to keep you energized:

- pH 9.5 alkaline water - I suggest you invest in a good quality alkaline filter to obtain this water, my blog has some further recommendations.
- Himalayan salt -it contains magnesium, iron and other vital minerals and you can use it to give your smoothies and soups more taste.
- Grasses- you can also use powdered grasses to save time, make sure you research the brand. I highly

recommend products from pH Miracle. You can order them from Amazon, or search for local distributors that sell them (since I live in Spain, I purchase mine from a local company, which makes it cheaper for me than ordering from the US). pH Miracle supplements are organic and great quality (you will experience their positive effects in your body sooner than you expect).

- Cucumber
- Kale
- Kelp
- Spinach (baby and grown)
- Parsley
- Broccoli
- All kinds of Sprouts (soy, alfalfa etc)
- Sea Vegetables (Kelp)

Again, if for some reason you can't find the ingredients, contact me here:

martaholisticwellness@gmail.com

I can help you change and personalize your recipes. I understand that, depending on your location, some ingredients may be difficult to find.

However, remember, you don't need all of the ingredients. Simply choose what you like and what you can find in your country/city. Use your imagination for blending them and creating your amazing alkaline drinks. Use this recipe book as a template.

JUICES OR SMOOTHIES?

One more tip - avoid fruit juices, with the exception of lemons, limes, grapefruits, and tomatoes. Most juices are pure sugar and no fiber. Focus on vegetable juices, instead. You can add fruits to your vegetable juices to taste and help make the transition.

Juicing is recommended to those who have a sensitive digestive system or illness that inhibits your body from processing fiber. Since there is no fiber, you only get nutrients, and your body does not need extra energy to digest it. This is why juicing vegetables first thing in the morning is so beneficial for your health, in addition to giving you a real energy boost.

Why you should avoid fruit juices (even homemade):

We already know that most fruits contain sugar, so imagine what happens when you juice them... When you remove the fiber, the liquid juice is absorbed into your blood stream much quicker than it does with fiber. This is why, if you are juicing fruits, it will lead to unstable blood sugar levels and a drop in blood sugar. This can cause low energy levels and sugar cravings. Drinking pure fruit juices will make you hungry, and your body will crave sugar to add to the vicious cycle...

Exception: If you have an occasional fruit juice, make sure you dilute it in some water..

Smoothies are a different story, because when you blend fruit, you also get fiber. So when you drink it, your body says 'no' to more when you are full. Fruit smoothies are a great component of the 20% acid part of your alkaline diet. They are natural, raw and nutritious.

Blending - yes, it's also good for you and smoothies will make you feel full longer. However, if you can't tolerate too much fiber because of any specific digestive problems, go for juicing first. Juice veggies and give your body more energy! As for fruit juices, choose alkaline non-sugary fruits (lemons, limes, grapefruits, pomegranates).

Now, it's time to put theory into practice...

Part 1 Alkaline Juices

Alkaline juices are the best energy boost you can get. Fiber-free and rich in nutrients, they are really easy to digest!

The Green Bomb Juice

Serves: 1-2

Ingredients:

- 1 cup fresh spinach
- 1 cup fresh kale
- 2 fresh cucumbers
- ½ green apple
- 2 carrots
- 2 cups fresh coconut water
- A few mint leaves
- Ice cubes

Instructions:

- ➤ Thoroughly wash the spinach and kale leaves.
- ➤ Place them in a bowl of cold water containing ice cubes.
- ➤ Meanwhile, cut the cucumber (or zucchini), carrots and green apple into small pieces.
- ➤ Juice the ingredients using a juicer (preferably low-speed, Omega juicers are great for that!)

- Place in a jar and add in some of the coconut water and stir until smooth.
- Chop the mint leaves roughly and mix it into the juice. They will flavor it in an incredible way! You can also throw in a few ice cubes.
- Your juice is ready to serve and is best consumed chilled.
- Enjoy, alkalize and energize!

8/10

39 calories for 250 ml rh. well worth it :)

Veggie Blast with a Twist

Serves: 3-4

Ingredients:

- 2 carrots
- 1 cup cabbage
- 1 cup fresh chives
- 1 cup fresh broccoli florets
- 1 cup fresh pumpkin, diced
- 1 cup radish
- 2 cups fresh coconut water
- 1 onion
- 2 garlic cloves
- Ice cubes
- Himalaya salt and pepper to taste

Instructions:

- ➢ Place the cabbage leaves in cold water containing ice cubes.
- ➢ Peel and cut the rest of the ingredients.
- ➢ Separate the broccoli into individual florets and wash it thoroughly under running water.
- ➢ Chop off the two ends of the radish and use a peeler to make thin slivers of it.
- ➢ Juice the ingredients using a juicer (preferably low-speed, Omega juicers are great for that!)

- Place your juice in a bowl or in a jar along with the coconut water and mix until well combined.
- Add Himalaya salt and pepper to taste.
- Garnish with radish slivers and serve.
- Enjoy!

Sweet Treat Veggie Juice

Serves: 3-4

Ingredients:

- 2 cups pomegranate seeds
- 1 cup sweet beetroot slices
- 1 cup cherry tomatoes
- ¼ cup watermelon
- 2 red bell peppers
- 2 cups fresh coconut water
- Ginger ice cubes (juice some ginger and freeze)
- 1 lemon, juiced
- Optional: stevia to sweeten

Instructions:

- ➤ Place the lemon juice in a small bowl.
- ➤ Deseed the pomegranate and place it in a bowl containing the lemon juice.
- ➤ Now, peel and cut the beetroot and the rest of the ingredients.
- ➤ Place the ingredients in a juicer. Juice well.
- ➤ Place in a bowl or a jar.
- ➤ Add in the coconut water and mix. Sweeten with stevia (optional).
- ➤ Pour in glasses and ginger ice cubes and serve.
- ➤ Enjoy!

Kale and Zucchini Juice Easy

Serves: 1

Ingredients:

- 2 cups zucchini slices
- 2 cups kale leaves
- 1 cup fresh radish
- 1 fresh turnip
- 1 cup alkaline water
- Ice cubes
- Stevia to sweeten

Instructions:

➤ Place the kale leaves in water containing ice after cleaning it under running water.
➤ Cut the zucchini into small pieces.
➤ Use a peeler to peel the skins of the radish and turnip and peel it further to make thin shavings.
➤ Place the zucchini, radish, kale and turnip in a juicer. Extract juice.
➤ Mix with 1 cup alkaline water and stevia to taste.
➤ Enjoy!

Coriander Coconut Cocktail

Serves: 1-2

Ingredients:

- 2 cups coriander leaves
- 2 tablespoons fresh mint leaves
- 2 cups coconut water
- 1 cup lemon juice
- Himalayan salt to taste
- ½ cup rocket leaves (aragula)
- Ice cubes

Instructions:

- Clean coriander and rocket thoroughly
- Place in a juicer and extract the juices. Set aside.
- Wash and mince mint leaves.
- Mix the green juice with lemon juice and coconut water
- Pour it into a glass and top with the Himalaya salt and mint.
- Serve chilled or with ice cubes added in if you wish.
- Enjoy!

Ginger Wheatgrass Medley

Serves: 2-4

Ingredients:

- 2 cups cucumber slices
- 1 cup wheat grass
- ¼ cup ginger slices
- Himalayan crystal salt
- Black pepper
- 1 cup coconut water
- 1 cup raw almond milk
- ¼ cup fresh mint leaves
- ½ cup lemon juice
- Ice cubes

Instructions:

- Wash all the greens
- Clean and peel the ginger
- Roughly chop it and place it in a juicer. Add cucumber slices and wheat grass. Extract their juices.
- Place in a jar.
- Add in some coconut water and almond milk and give it an energetic mix until smooth.

➢ Serve with the mint leaves on top. Season with black pepper and Himalaya salt if you wish. Add ice cubes.

➢ Enjoy!

Lemon and Beet Easy Drink

Serves: 1-2

Ingredients:

- 1 cup lemon grass
- ½ cup lime juice
- 1 cup grapefruit juice (approx. 3 big grapefruits)
- 2 cups beetroot slices
- 2 tablespoons minced chives
- 2 cups sweet potato slices
- 1 green apple
- Fresh parsley leaves
- Ice cubes

Instructions:

- ➢ Wash, peel and chop all the ingredients.
- ➢ Place the sweet potatoes in a juicer. Add beetroot, lemon grass, apple and chives.
- ➢ Extract their juices and pour in a jar.
- ➢ Add in the lime juice and the grapefruit juice and mix until well combined.
- ➢ Serve with a sprinkling of fresh parsley on top and ice cubes, if desired.
- ➢ Enjoy!

Ayurvedic Cleanser Mega Juice

Ingredients:

- 1 tablespoon cumin powder
- Himalayan salt
- 1 teaspoon pepper
- 1 cup alkaline water (slightly warm but not hot)
- ½ cup lemon juice
- 1 teaspoon turmeric powder
- Fresh cilantro leaves
- Ginger ice cubes (juice and freeze some ginger into ice cubes)

Instructions:

➢ To prepare the cleanser, mix the alkaline water with the lemon juice and give it a good mix.

➢ Add 1 tablespoon of cumin powder and mix until at least half of it dissolves.

➢ Top it with the fresh parsley leaves and a sprinkling of 1 teaspoon turmeric powder.

➢ Add a pinch of Himalaya salt and black pepper.

➢ This drink can be had twice a week for full body cleansing.

Fennel Magic Alka-Juice

Serves: 1-2

Ingredients:

- 2 cups fennel, chopped
- 2 tablespoons fennel seeds + 1 divided
- 2 cups spinach
- 2 cups carrot slices
- 1 pear, peeled and sliced
- ½ cup lemon juice
- Ice cubes

Instructions:

- ➢ Wash all ingredients well. Clean and chop.
- ➢ Add all ingredients (fennel, spinach, carrots, pear) through juicer.
- ➢ Mix in some lemon juice. Place in a tall glass
- ➢ Serve with a sprinkling of fennel seeds on top and it is best served chilled.
- ➢ Ice cubes, and ginger ice cubes work great with this juice.
- ➢ Enjoy!

Kelp and Garlic Alkalyzer

Serves: 1-2

Ingredients:

- 2 cups fresh kelp
- 1 cup broccoli florets
- 4 big tomatoes, peeled and sliced
- 2 garlic cloves
- 1 sweet potato
- 1 teaspoon Himalayan crystal salt
- Ice cubes
- Black pepper

Instructions:

- ➢ Wash, peel and chop all the ingredients as required.
- ➢ Cut the potato into small pieces.
- ➢ Add all ingredients through juicer.
- ➢ Pour the juice into a glass and top it with the garlic, black pepper and salt mix.
- ➢ Enjoy!

Celery Coconut Infusion

Serves: 2-3

Ingredients:

- 2 cups celery
- 2 cups spinach leaves
- 2 cups parsley leaves
- 2 cups coconut water
- 1 cup carrot
- Ice cubes

Instructions:

- ➤ Clean the spinach thoroughly and place it in a bowl of water containing ice cubes.
- ➤ Clean the celery and parsley and place in a blender along with the spinach and finely chopped carrot.
- ➤ Add in the coconut water and blend until smooth. If you are using a juicer, then first juice the veggies and then mix with some chilled coconut water.
- ➤ Serve with ice cubes if you wish.
- ➤ Enjoy!

Cantaloupe Grapefruit Mix

Serves: 1-2

Ingredients:

- 2 grapefruits, juiced
- 2 cucumbers, peeled and sliced
- 1 big zucchini, peeled and sliced
- 2 lemons, juiced
- ½ cup cantaloupe, rind removed
- 1 cup alkaline water
- 2 cups pumpkin
- Ice cubes

Instructions:

➢ First squeeze lemons and grapefruits. Strain if necessary. Set the juice aside.

➢ Chop cantaloupe and pumpkin into small pieces.

➢ Place them in a juicer. Add zucchini and cucumber slices. Juice.

➢ Combine with the lemon and grapefruit juice. Add some alkaline water if you wish.

➢ Sweeten with stevia if you wish and serve!

➢ Add ice cubes or ginger ice cubes.

➢ Enjoy!

Sweet Grapefruit Easy Mix

Pressed for time and want to alkalize? This recipe is super easy and full of alkalinity!

Serves: 1-2

Ingredients:

- 2 grapefruits
- 1 cup coconut water
- 1 cup almond milk
- ½ lemon
- 1 teaspoon powdered ginger
- ¼ cup warm water (not boiling)

Instructions:

➢ Combine the powdered ginger and warm water until dissolved.
➢ Add the lemon and grapefruit juice.
➢ Add the coconut water and almond milk.
➢ Add ice cubes or ginger ice cubes.
➢ Enjoy!

ok quite refreshing

not a wow but ok

6/10.

150 cal not worth it

Alkaline Energy on a Budget Juice

I have noticed that many people are put off by alkaline juices and drinks, as they imagine that it's something extremely expensive and that most ingredients are difficult to get. To some extent this is true - certain exotic ingredients and alkaline supplements are pricey, but you don't need all of them. Learn how to make use of what you already have in your kitchen. This is an amazing alkaline drink, that you can have slightly warm (in the winter) or chilled and with ice cubes. You don't even need a juicer!

Serves: 2

Ingredients:

- 1 cup of mint infusion, cooled down
- 1 cup raw almond milk
- Juice of 1 orange
- Juice of 2 lemons
- Optional: ¼ cup warm water

Instructions:

➢ Mix all the ingredients.
➢ Add some warm water on top and mix again- this will stimulate digestion.

➢ Optional: instead of warm water, you can add in some ice cubes. It's up to you!

➢ Enjoy!

Warming Up Alkaline Juice

This juice balances your pH and strengthens your immune system. Drink it regularly and you will never catch a cold again!

Serves: 1-2

Ingredients:

- 1 cup rosemary infusion, cooled
- 1 cup thyme infusion, cooled
- 2 lemons
- 2 apples
- ½ cup of ginger slices
- 2 garlic cloves, peeled

Instructions:

➢ First, make rosemary and thyme infusion and set aside to cool down. They should be slightly warm, but not boiling.
➢ Now, juice lemons, apples, ginger and garlic.
➢ Place rosemary-thyme infusion in a big glass or a jar. Add juiced ingredients and stir well.
➢ Drink slightly warm. Add a bit of organic, raw honey if you wish.

➢ Enjoy!

My tip- juice ginger and freeze it as ginger ice cubes- ready to serve with your juices, smoothies and teas.

Coconut Spicy Juice

Serves: 2

Ingredients:

- 2 cups coconut milk
- Juice of 2 limes
- 2 cups of spinach, washed and dried
- ½ cup ginger slices, peeled
- 2 garlic cloves, peeled
- 1 turnip (keep the long bunch of its green head), chopped
- Pinch of Cinnamon powder

Instructions:

- First combine spinach, ginger, turnip and garlic in a juicer. Extract their juice.
- Using a jar, combine the fresh juice with coconut milk.
- Add lime juice and mix well.
- Top with cinnamon powder.
- Enjoy!

Amazing Skin Juice

Drink one glass (or more) of this amazing anti-age juice a day, and you will have beautiful skin.

Serves: 1

Ingredients:

- 4 big tomatoes
- 2 cucumbers, sliced
- 1 cup broccoli florets
- 2 carrots, sliced
- A handful fresh mint leaves
- Himalaya salt to taste

Instructions:

- Wash all ingredients well.
- Add all ingredients through juicer.
- Add some Himalaya salt.
- Serve and enjoy!

Citrus Rooibos Ice Tea Style Juice

This is a really quick recipe and you don't need a juicer or a blender to make it.

Serves: 2

Ingredients:

- 1 cup of rooibos tea, cooled
- 1 cup alkaline water
- 2 grapefruits
- 1 lime
- 1 lemon
- Stevia

Instructions:

➢ Squeeze lemon, lime and grapefruits.
➢ In a jar, combine the juice with rooibos tea.
➢ Add some stevia to sweeten. Stevia is alkaline. Alternatively you can use some raw organic honey (honey is not alkaline).
➢ Add some ice cubes (ginger ice cubes are great with this recipe) and serve.
➢ Enjoy!

Green, Warm Milk Juice

I love this recipe in the winter. It warms me up and keeps my belly happy. I don't know about you, but I only like cold drinks in the summer. This super alkaline drink is now my favourite coffee replacement. It gives me incredible energy!

Serves: 2

Ingredients:

- 2 cups raw almond milk
- 2 cups spinach
- 2 cups kale
- ½ cup ginger slices
- 2 garlic cloves, peeled
- 1 cucumber, peeled and sliced
- 1 lime, juiced

Instructions:

- Warm up the almond milk and set aside.
- In the meantime, extract the juice from all other ingredients (kale, spinach, ginger, garlic and cucumber).
- Now, combine the fresh green juice with warm, almond milk.
- Stir well. Add lime juice.

- Sprinkle some cinnamon powder on top.
- If you are really pressed for time, you might consider purchasing some powdered greens. They are real time savers!
- Enjoy and energize!

Simple Tomato Delight Juice

Could I live without cilantro? The answer is no. Ever since I discovered it, I got hooked on it. It gives my food and drinks an incredible flavour!

Serves: 2

Ingredients:

- ½ cup fresh cilantro
- 1 cup spinach
- 4 big tomatoes
- 1 cup coconut water, chilled
- Himalaya salt to taste

Instructions:

1. First wash cilantro, spinach and tomatoes.
2. Peel tomatoes and place them in a juicer, add the greens.
3. Extract juices and mix it with some fresh coconut water.
4. Add some Himalaya salt if you wish.
5. Enjoy!

Part 2 Alkaline Smoothies

Rhubarb and Avocado Satisfying Smoothie

Serves: 2

Ingredients:

- 2 cups rhubarb
- 2 avocados
- 2 cups coconut water
- 2 tablespoons lemon juice
- 1 cup almond milk, raw
- 1 tablespoon coconut oil
- 1 teaspoon cinnamon

Instructions:

- Clean and place the rhubarb in boiling water. Leave for 5 minutes. Drain and set aside.
- Meanwhile, deseed the avocado and scoop out the flesh.
- Place the avocado flesh in blender. Add coconut water, almond milk and rhubarb.
- Blend until smooth.
- Add in the lemon juice, cinnamon and coconut milk.
- Place it in a glass and serve. Garnish with a slice of lemon.
- Enjoy!

Avocado Surprise Blend

Serves: 2-3

Ingredients:

- 2 avocados
- 2 tablespoons lemon juice
- Pinch of Himalayan crystal salt
- 2 cups fresh coconut water
- 1 cup fresh fig
- Fresh mint leaves
- Ice cubes

Instructions:

- ➤ Use a spoon to scoop out the flesh from the avocado.
- ➤ Add in the lemon juice and salt and mix well.
- ➤ Peel the skin of the figs (optional).Place the fig in the blender along with the coconut and the avocado and blend until smooth.
- ➤ Add more coconut water or ice until you get the consistency you like.
- ➤ Serve with a sprinkling of fresh mint leaves on top.
- ➤ Enjoy!

Cabbage and Endive Energy Drink

Serves: 2-3

Ingredients:

- 2 cups cabbage
- 2 cups endive
- 1 tablespoon sesame seeds
- 1 tablespoon sunflower seeds
- 2 avocados
- 1 tablespoon lime juice
- ½ cup pumpkin slices
- Pinch of Himalayan crystal salt
- 1 cup distilled alkaline water
- 2 cups coconut water
- Ice cubes
- Coconut cream

Instructions:

- ➤ Place the cabbage leaves in cold water containing ice cubes.
- ➤ You can do the same with the endives after it has been washed thoroughly under a running tap.
- ➤ Place the sunflower and sesame seeds in a small pan and heat it on low for a few minutes. Set aside to cool.
- ➤ Chop the pumpkin into small pieces.

- ➢ Use a spoon to scoop out the flesh from the avocado and place it in a blender.
- ➢ Add the ingredients one at a time and blend until smooth.
- ➢ Mix the liquid with the coconut water.
- ➢ Add some coconut cream and seeds on top.
- ➢ Enjoy!

Spicy Creamy Smoothie
Serves: 2

Ingredients:

- 2 cups coconut flesh
- 2 cups coconut cream
- 2 tablespoons cinnamon powder
- 1 tablespoon clove powder
- 1 teaspoon cayenne pepper
- 1 teaspoon ginger powder
- 1 teaspoon garlic powder
- 1 teaspoon cumin powder
- 1 teaspoon coriander powder
- A pinch of Himalayan crystal salt

Instructions:

- ➤ Place the coconut flesh and coconut water in a blender and blend until fully smooth and creamy.
- ➤ Heat all of the spices on a very low flame for 10 minutes. Keep a close eye on these. Place the coconut mix in a glass and stir in 2 tablespoons of the spice mix into it.
- ➤ Sprinkle some salt on top and serve chilled.
- ➤ Enjoy!

Nutty Naughty Smoothie

This smoothie gives me energy before strenuous workouts. I can run miles!!!

Serves: 1-2

Ingredients:

- 2 tablespoons flax seeds
- 2 tablespoons sesame seeds
- 2 tablespoons pumpkin seeds
- 2 tablespoons sunflower seeds
- 5 tablespoons almonds
- 2 cups coconut cream
- 1 cup coconut water
- 1 cup coconut flesh
- A pinch of Himalayan crystal salt

Instructions:

➢ Place the flax seeds, sesame seeds, pumpkin seeds, sunflower seeds in a small pan and heat it on low for a few minutes. Keep an eye on it to prevent burning.

➢ Place the coconut flesh and water in the blender and blend until it is smooth.

➢ Remove the seeds from the pan and blend to make a coarse powder.

- Chop the almonds roughly and place it in the same pan. Blend.
- Mix the nut and seed mixture with the coconut flesh mix.
- Heat on low for 5 minutes to help release the nutty flavor.
- Place a spoon full of the coconut cream on top and sprinkle the almonds over it to serve.
- Enjoy!

Lemon Avocado Alka-Smoothie

Serves: 2

Ingredients:

- 2 lemons, juiced
- 2 avocados
- 1 lime
- 2 cups coconut flesh
- 1 cup coconut water
- 1 teaspoon Himalayan crystal salt
- 2 tablespoons Udo's oil
- 2 tablespoons olive oil
- Ice cubes

Instructions:

- Peel the lime and chop into small pieces. Set aside.
- Deseed the avocado and scoop all the flesh out.
- Place it in the blender along with the ice cubes, coconut flesh and coconut water and blend until completely smooth.
- Add in the Udo's oil and the olive oil and allow it to mix.
-
- Serve with lime and a pinch of Himalayan salt sprinkled on top.

Betroot Smoothie

This smoothie will keep your belly full and prevent food cravings.

Serves: 2

Ingredients:

- 2 carrots
- 2 cups beetroots, sliced
- 1 cup tofu, diced (you can also use quinoa). If you are Paleo, choose avocados instead.
- 3 tablespoons lemon juice
- Pinch of Himalayan crystal salt
- 1 teaspoon pepper
- 2 tablespoons avocado oil
- 5 tablespoons fresh pomegranate seeds
- 2 tablespoons ginger
- Mint leaves to sprinkle
- Ice cubes
- Alkaline water (about 1 cup)
- Coconut water (about 1 cup)

Instructions:

- ➢ Chop the carrots and beetroots. Place the slices in a bowl containing 2 tablespoons of lemon juice and salt.
- ➢ In another bowl add in one tablespoon of lemon juice, pepper and pomegranate seeds along with the mint leaves.
- ➢ While that soaks, place the tofu in a blender along with the avocado oil and ginger and blend until creamy.
- ➢ (Optional)Add distilled alkaline water or coconut water for better consistency.
- ➢ Add the other ingredients and blend until smooth. Add it to the coconut mix and blend until well combined.
- ➢ Place it in a glass and sprinkle the pomegranate and mint. Serve.
- ➢ Enjoy!

Basil Coconut Smoothie

Serves: 2-4

Ingredients:

- 2 cups fresh basil leaves
- 2 cups fresh mint leaves
- 2 cups almond milk
- 1 cup coconut water
- 1 cup coconut cream
- 2 tablespoons flax seed oil
- 2 tablespoons coconut oil
- 2 tablespoons cilantro leaves
- Ice cubes

Instructions:

- Thoroughly cleanse the basil and mint leaves and place in boiling water for 2 minutes. Strain, but set water aside.
- Place the almond milk and coconut cream in a blender and blend until completely smooth.
- Place the leaves in a blender along with the coconut water and blend until smooth.
- Add the coconut flesh, flax seed oil, and ice cubes to the blender. Blend until smooth.
- Mix this with the mint water and coconut oil. Place it in a glass.

➢ Serve with some fresh cilantro on top.

➢ Enjoy!

Squash Olive Smoothie

Olives are actually acidic, but no worries. The Alkaline Diet is not about eating 100% alkaline foods. Remember the 20/80 rule. It means that while 80% of your diet should be composed of alkaline foods, the remaining 20% can be acidic. Of course, make sure that you eat wholesome, natural and organic foods.

Serves:3-4

Ingredients:

- 2 cups squash
- 2 cups zucchini slices
- 1 cup fresh olives (green)
- 5 tablespoons olive oil (intense taste option is a better choice)
- 2 cups celery
- 1/2 teaspoon Himalayan crystal salt
- 2 tablespoon lemon juice
- 1 cup coconut flesh
- 1 cup coconut water
- 2 tablespoons sesame seeds
- Ice cubes

Instructions:

➢ Chop the squash and zucchini into small pieces and place it in the bowl containing salt and lemon juice.

- Meanwhile, pit the olives and chop it into small pieces.
- Place the olives in a blender along with the squash, zucchini, celery and coconut water and blend it until completely smooth.
- Add in the olive oil and coconut flesh and blend again.
- Toast the sesame seeds on a low flame until golden.
- Place the ice cubes in a glass and pour the smoothie on top.
- Sprinkle the sesame seeds on top and serve.
- Enjoy!

Carrot and Sprout Smoothie

Serves: 4

Ingredients:

- 2 cups carrot slices
- 2 cups bean sprouts (skip this step if you follow the Paleo Diet)
- 2 cups coconut flesh
- 2 cups coconut cream
- 1 cup sweet potato
- 1 cup coconut water
- 2 tablespoons Udo's oil
- 2 tablespoons olive oil
- Himalaya salt to taste
- Black pepper to taste

Instructions:

- Thoroughly cleanse the bean sprouts. Boil them to soften.
- Chop the sweet potato into small pieces and boil until soft. Let cool.
- Place the coconut cream and flesh in a blender and blend until smooth.
- Add in the Udo's oil gradually to combine.
- Add in the olive oil in the same way and set it aside.

- ➤ Place the coconut water, chopped carrot, sweet potato and sprouts pieces in the blender and blend until smooth.
- ➤ Place the mixture in a glass and mix in 2 to 3 tablespoons of the coconut cream.
- ➤ Use Himalaya salt and black pepper to taste.
- ➤ Enjoy. It's delicious and nutritious! You can have it warm or chilled. It will keep you full, happy and energized!

Asparagus Tomato Smoothie

Serves: 2-3

Ingredients:

- 2 cups asparagus
- 1/8 cup wakame seaweed
- 2 tomatoes, peeled
- 1 cup coconut water
- 2 cups coconut milk
- Himalayan crystal salt
- 2 tablespoons pumpkin seeds

Instructions:

- ➤ Place wakame seaweed in warm water for 5 minutes.
- ➤ Clean asparagus and place it in boiling water
- ➤ Once it softens, allow it to cool over the counter.
- ➤ Chop the tomatoes into small pieces and place them in a blender.
- ➤ Add the asparagus and wakame.
- ➤ Blend and place in a bowl.
- ➤ Season with Himalaya salt and pepper.
- ➤ Add in the coconut water, salt and coconut milk and give it a good mix.
- ➤ Heat the pumpkin seeds in a pan. Allow them to cool. Chop them roughly to sprinkle over the smoothie.
- ➤ Enjoy! This is pure alkalinity!

Pomegranate Mint Smoothie

Serves: 2

Ingredients:

- 2 cups pomegranate seeds
- 2 cups mint leaves
- 1 cup coconut water
- 2 cups coconut cream
- 1 teaspoon Himalayan salt
- Ice cubes

Instructions:

- ➤ Place one cup of the pomegranate seeds in boiling water for 2 minutes and switch off the heat.
- ➤ Place the ice cubes, mint leaves, coconut cream and the rest of the pomegranate seeds in the blender and blend until completely smooth.
- ➤ Strain the pomegranate water and mix it with the coconut water.
- ➤ Combine the mixtures and pour into a tall glass.
- ➤ Sprinkle some of the salt crystals on top and serve.
- ➤ Enjoy!

Wakame Coconut Smoothie

Serves: 2

Ingredients:

- 1/4 cup dry Wakame seaweed
- 1 cups spinach
- 2 cups cabbage
- 1 cup coconut flesh
- 2 cups coconut cream
- 2 cups coconut water
- 1 tablespoon Udo's oil
- A few banana slices to taste
- Ice cubes
- cinnamon

Instructions:

- ➢ Thoroughly cleanse the Wakame leaves and place in warm water to soften.
- ➢ Clean the cabbage and spinach leaves and place in cold water containing ice cubes.
- ➢ Place the coconut cream and flesh in the blender and blend until smooth.
- ➢ Add in the Udo's oil gradually and allow it to mix well.
- ➢ Add in the ice cubes and blend.

- ➢ Place the mixture in a bowl.
- ➢ Now place the Wakame, cabbage, banana slices and spinach in the blender along with the coconut water and blend.
- ➢ Combine the two mixtures..
- ➢ Serve in a tall glass with some cinnamon sprinkled on top.
- ➢ Enjoy! Wakame is a bomb of alkaline minerals that your body really needs!

Grapefruit and Lemon Smoothie

Serves: 2-3

Ingredients:

- 2 lemons, juiced
- 1 lime
- 2 grapefruits
- 2 cups coconut water
- 1 tablespoon coconut oil
- 5 tablespoon almonds
- 1 teaspoon stevia

Instructions:

- Mix the lemon juice and coconut water.
- Place in a fridge.
- Meanwhile, place the almonds in a pan to brown on a low flame and chop the lime into tiny pieces.
- Use a spoon to scoop out all the flesh from the grapefruit. Blend.
- Add in some stevia and coconut oil and blend.
- Mix in the coconut and lemon water.
- Sprinkle some almonds and lime over it and serve. This smoothie is great as a dessert.
- Enjoy!

Simple Cabbage Smoothie

Serves: 2

Ingredients:

- 2 cups cabbage
- ¼ cup coconut cream
- 1 cup almond milk
- A few banana slices to taste
- 1 teaspoon coconut oil
- Ice cubes
- Cinnamon

Instructions:

- ➢ Clean and dry the cabbage leaves
- ➢ Place all the ingredients (aside from coconut oil) in a blender and blend until smooth.
- ➢ Now add in some coconut oil and mix well.
- ➢ Add some ice cubes if you wish.
- ➢ Serve in a tall glass.
- ➢ Sprinkle over some cinnamon on top and garnish with a slice of lemon.
- ➢ Enjoy! Cabbage can be so nice!

Barley Water Smoothie

Serves: 2-3

Ingredients:

- 1 cup almond milk
- 1 cup barley grains (skip if you are Paleo)
- 2 cups fresh coconut flesh
- 1 avocado
- 1 tablespoon coconut oil
- 2 tablespoons dates
- A few raisins
- Ice cubes

Instructions:

- ➤ Place barley in a bowl of hot water.
- ➤ Add some dates and raisins and let them soak in. Set aside.
- ➤ Cut and deseed the avocado.
- ➤ Scoop the flesh of the avocado out and place it in a blender.
- ➤ Add in the ice cubes, almond milk, and the coconut flesh and blend. Mix in coconut oil.
- ➤ Then, strain the dates and barley, place in blender and blend until smooth.

- ➤ Add some barley water to achieve desired consistency.
- ➤ Pour it in a tall glass and serve.
- ➤ Enjoy! This is a great breakfast smoothie!

Wheat Grass and Papaya Smoothie

Serves: 2

Ingredients:

- 2 cups wheat grass, juiced
- 2 teaspoons sea kelp powder (optional)
- 2 cups coconut water
- 2 tablespoons Udo's oil
- 2 tablespoons dates
- 2 cups of papaya slices
- Cinnamon
- Ice cubes

Instructions:

➤ Place the dates in boiling water and allow it to soften completely.

➤ Juice wheat grass and set aside. Wheat grass can be also used directly in a smoothie, but I prefer to juice it and then add it to my smoothie (it's easier to digest juiced).

➤ Chop the dates and papaya.

➤ Blend the coconut water, dates, papaya and Udo's oil until creamy.

➤ Add wheat grass juice, kelp powder and mix again.

➤ Pour it into a tall glass and sprinkle some cinnamon and nutmeg powder on top. Enjoy!

Chili Pepper Smoothie

Serves: 3

Ingredients:

- 1 big red bell pepper
- 1 cup spinach
- 1 cup celery, chopped
- 2 cups coconut flesh
- 1/2 cup coconut cream
- 2 cups coconut water
- 1 teaspoon Himalayan salt
- 1 teaspoon pepper powder
- 1 tablespoon Udo's oil
- 1 teaspoon olive oil
- 1 teaspoon chili powder
- Ice cubes
- Optional: some finely chopped jalapenos

Instructions:

➢ Clean the celery leaves and place in a steamer or boiling water to help soften it for 5 minutes. Wash the spinach and other ingredients.

- ➤ Place the coconut cream and flesh in a blender and blend until smooth. Add in the bell pepper, spinach, celery and coconut water. Blend again.
- ➤ Add in the Udo's oil gradually and allow it to come together.
- ➤ Add in the ice cubes, olive oil, chili powder and the salt and mix.
- ➤ Serve it in a tall glass with some salt sprinkled on top and if you like it spicy, then you can sprinkle some finely chopped jalapenos as well.
- ➤ Enjoy!

*My tip- you can serve it with some quinoa! This smoothie can be made thicker so that you use it as a cream or soup.

Anti-Hangover Orange Alka Smoothie

Suffering from a self-inflicted illness called "hangover"? Try this smoothie and balance your pH levels immediately. I wish someone had told me this when I was a college student!

Serves: 2

Ingredients:

- 2 oranges, juiced
- 2 lemons, juiced
- 1 cup alkaline water
- 4 carrots
- 4 tomatoes, peeled
- 1 garlic clove
- Stevia to sweeten (optional)
- Optional: green powders (alfalfa or grasses)

Instructions:

- Peel and cut the carrots and tomatoes.
- Place them in a blender. Add garlic, lemon juice and orange juice. Blend.
- Add some alkaline water and mix well. Sweeten with stevia. Add your green powders if you wish. (Alfalfa is a great option - it is full of minerals.)
- Serve immediately. It works- trust me!

Alkaline Curry Gazpacho Smoothie

This recipe is inspired by Spanish Gazpacho, however I have removed vinegar (vinegar is acid forming) and used other ingredients instead.

Curry and coconut milk give it a nice, oriental taste.

Serves: 1-2

Ingredients:

- 4 tomatoes
- 2 cucumbers
- Half of red pepper
- 1 garlic clove
- Half cup of almond milk
- 1 tablespoon of olive oil (cold-pressed, organic)
- Pinch of Himalaya salt
- Pinch of black pepper
- Pinch of curry
- A few green olives
- 2 tablespoons of coconut milk (or cream)

Instructions:

- ➢ Wash, peel and cut the cucumbers, pepper and tomatoes.
- ➢ Place them in a blender.

- ➤ Add garlic cloves, green olives and almond milk. Blend until smooth.
- ➤ Stir well and add Himalaya salt, pepper and curry.
- ➤ Add olive oil and stir again.
- ➤ Add coconut cream or milk on top. Garnish with a slice of cucumber.
- ➤ Serve immediately, enjoy!

Sweet Alkaline Dream

Here's another delicious alkaline drink, made of 100% alkaline ingredients.

Serves: 2

Ingredients:

- 1 cup of coconut milk
- 1 cup of almond milk
- 1 teaspoon of nutmeg
- 1 teaspoon of clove
- 1 teaspoon of cinnamon
- Juice of 2 lemons
- 1 tablespoon of chia seeds
- 1 avocado, peeled, pitted

Instructions:

- Bring almond milk, nutmeg and clove to a boil. Turn off the heat and cover.
- Allow the almond milk infusion to cool.
- Blend avocado, coconut milk, chia seeds and lemon juice using a blender.
- Combine with the almond milk infusion.
- Sprinkle over some cinnamon.
- Enjoy!

OPTIONAL:

You can add some green powder (alfalfa, green grasses, or any other quality alkaline product of your choice).

Oat Grass and Ginger Smoothie

Serves: 2

Ingredients:

- 2 cups oat grass , juiced
- 1 lemon, juiced
- ¼ cup ginger slices
- 2 cups coconut water
- 2 cucumbers, peeled and sliced
- 1 avocado
- 1 tablespoon olive oil
- 1/2 cup coconut milk
- Stevia to sweeten
- Ice cubes

Instructions:

- ➢ Blend the coconut water, lemon juice, cucumbers, avocado and ice cubes until smooth.
- ➢ Pour in the fresh oat grass juice. Mix well.
- ➢ Add coconut milk and stevia to sweeten.
- ➢ Serve immediately!

Alfalfa Green Smoothie

Serves: 2

Ingredients:

- 2 cups raw almond milk
- 2 tablespoons alfalfa powder
- 1 green apple
- A few kale leaves
- 1 garlic clove, peeled
- 1/8 cup sesame powder
- ¼ cup pumpkin seeds (soaked in water for at least a few hours)

Instructions:

- ➢ Wash apple and kale. Peel and chop the apple.
- ➢ Place apple and kale in a blender along with the garlic clove, sesame powder, pumpkin seeds and almond milk.
- ➢ Blend well. Now add alfalfa powder, stir in and blend again.
- ➢ Serve immediately. It's pure energy your body needs so much!

Part 3 Alkaline Teas and Infusions

Pepper Mint Tea Surprise

Serves: 2

Ingredients:

- 1 cup peppermint
- 1 cup regular mint
- 1 cup basil
- 2 tablespoons dates
- 0.5 liter alkaline water

Instructions:

- ➢ Boil water.
- ➢ Remove a ladle full of the water and pour it over the dates.
- ➢ Place the dates in a blender and make a puree out of it.
- ➢ Meanwhile, place the peppermint, mint and basil leaves in a blender and blend until smooth.
- ➢ Add the hot water to the mint mix and combine until mint is dissolved (approximately 5-15 minutes).
- ➢ To serve, pour the water through a sieve into a glass and mix in a teaspoon of the date puree.

Chamomile Tea with Parsley

Serves: 2

Ingredients:

- 2 cups chamomile flowers
- 2 cups parsley
- 2 cups (0.5 liter) alkaline water
- 2 tablespoons dates
- 2 tablespoons mint

Instructions:

- ➤ Boil the water.
- ➤ Add a ladle full to the dates and set it aside.
- ➤ Place the dates in a blender and blend to make a thick puree.
- ➤ Clean the chamomile thoroughly and roughly chop.
- ➤ Clean the parsley thoroughly and chop roughly.
- ➤ Place both the chamomile and parsley in a bowl and pour the boiling water on top.
- ➤ Allow it to stand for 15 to 20 minutes and then strain the liquid.
- ➤ Place the liquid back on the heat for 10 minutes.
- ➤ Pour the tea in a mug and mix in a tablespoon of the date puree.
- ➤ Sprinkle some mint leaves on top and serve.

➤ Chamomile has amazing health benefits and helps beat insomnia. Enjoy!

Lavender and Mint Tea

Serves: 2-3

Ingredients:

- 2 cups lavender flowers
- 2 cups mint leaves
- 3 cups distilled alkaline water

Instructions:

➤ Clean the lavender flowers thoroughly under running water.

➤ Chop it roughly and place it in a large saucepan.

➤ Clean and roughly chop the mint leaves and add to the sauce pan.

➤ Add the water to the pan and allow it to come to a boil.

➤ Once it starts to boil, lower the heat and simmer for 5 minutes.

➤ Strain and pour into a mug.

➤ Your lavender mint tea is ready to serve.

➤ Lavender has various properties in terms of protecting mental health. It is used to help chase away depression and also helps in bringing about mental peace. I call it, holistic wellness self-care!

Almond Milk and Rosemary Tea

Serves: 2

Ingredients:

- 2 cups almond milk
- 4 whole sprigs rosemary
- 2 tablespoons dates
- 2 tablespoons sago balls
- 1 tablespoon almond butter

Instructions:

- ➢ Heat the almond milk and rosemary in a saucepan.
- ➢ Once it comes to a boil, lower the heat.
- ➢ Allow it to simmer for 10 minutes.
- ➢ Add some hot water to the dates and set it aside.
- ➢ Heat the almond butter in a small pan and add in the sago balls.
- ➢ Once it starts to brown, turn off the heat.
- ➢ Puree the dates in a blender.
- ➢ Raise the heat of the almond milk and allow the rosemary to infuse completely.
- ➢ Switch off the heat and strain the milk. Add in the almond butter and sago balls mixture,
- ➢ Add in a tablespoon of the dates and mix.
- ➢ Enjoy!

Ayurvedic Alkaline Healing Tea

Serves: 2

Ingredients:

- 1 cup lemon juice
- 5 tablespoons ginger
- 2 tablespoons cardamom
- 1 tablespoon clove
- 4 cups alkaline water
- 2 tablespoons mint leaves

Instructions:

➢ Place water in a pot and allow it to come to a boil.
➢ Clean the ginger thoroughly and peel it.
➢ The ginger must be fresh and tender.
➢ Chop it roughly and place it in the boiling water.
➢ Meanwhile, place the clove and the cardamom in a small pan and heat to release its flavor.
➢ Grind the clove and cardamom using a mortar and pestle.
➢ If you don't have a mortar pestle then you can use a coffee grinder or place the spices in a Ziploc bag and crush using a rolling pin.
➢ Strain the ginger water and place it in a bowl.

- ➤ Add the lemon juice to it and mix.
- ➤ Top the tea with the clove and cardamom mix.
- ➤ Garnish with mint leaves and serve.
- ➤ This tea is great for coughs and colds and also helps strengthen immunity if consumed regularly.

Pumpkin and Flax Infusion Tea

Serves: 2

Ingredients:

- 2 cups pumpkin seeds
- 2 cups flax seeds
- 2 cups alkaline water
- 2 tablespoons mint leaves
- 2 tablespoons parsley leaves
- 2 tablespoons chives
- 1 teaspoon Himalayan crystal salt
- Construction paper
- Needle
- Thread
- Scissors

Instructions:

- Place the pumpkin and flax seeds in a small pan to brown on low heat.
- Meanwhile, chop the mint, parsley and chives roughly after washing thoroughly and pat it dry.
- Spread the herb mixture on a plate and place under full sun for at least an hour.(If you have a dehydrator, then you can use that instead or simply place it in an oven or microwave at 120 degrees for 10 minutes)

- The leaves will dry up like tea leaves and you can use them to brew tea.
- Place the two types of seeds in a blender and make a coarse powder.
- Cut out squares of construction paper.
- Place all ingredients, of an equal ratio, onto the paper.
- You can attach a string and use a stapler to fasten it.
- To prepare the tea, place the bag in a mug and pour hot distilled alkaline water over it.
- Dip the bag for 5 minutes and consume.

Rosehip and Lemon Tea

Serves: 2-3

Ingredients:

- 2 cups lemon juice
- 2 cups fresh rosehip
- 3 cups distilled alkaline water
- 2 tablespoons dates

Instructions:

- ➢ Boil water.
- ➢ Thoroughly clean the rosehips and remove all its seeds and tops.
- ➢ Halve each of them and add to the boiling water.
- ➢ Boil for 10 minutes. Strain.
- ➢ Make a puree out of the dates and mix it with the lemon juice.
- ➢ Fill half the glass with the lemon mix and the rest with the rosehip water.
- ➢ Serve hot or place it in the fridge to make it iced tea.

Yerba Mate and Mint Infusion Tea

I used to be a coffee person and so quitting caffeine was a big challenge for me. While yerba mate is not 100% alkaline (it contains caffeine, and caffeine is acidic), it is full of antioxidants. It also helps stimulate weight loss. I use yerba mate as well as green tea occasionally. If you are a coffee addict wanting to kick your habit, you might notice headaches. This is why, I suggest you use green tea or yerba mate to help you transition. Mix it with other herbs to balance it (herbs are alkaline).

Ever since a friend of mine, originally from Argentina, introduced me to yerba mate, I fell in love with it!

Enjoy!

Serves: 2-3

Ingredients:

- 2 tablespoons yerba mate
- 2-3 cups alkaline water
- 2 tablespoons mint

Instructions:

- ➢ Place the water in a pot and allow it to simmer.
- ➢ Make sure that it does not boil.
- ➢ Place the yerba mate in a glass.
- ➢ Add in the mint leaves and mix.
- ➢ Add the 5 tablespoons of warm water to it and allow the leaves to rise up. Wait a few minutes.
- ➢ Keep the temperature of the water around 170 F (75 Celsius).
- ➢ Now, pour the rest of the water into the glass and allow it to stand for a few minutes.
- ➢ Pour the tea through a strainer and serve warm.
- ➢ Remember to not use boiling water for this recipe as it can cause the yerba mate to go bitter.
- ➢ Yerba mate is a great digestive and can be had after a heavy meal. It is also quite rich in antioxidants and helps you maintain vibrant health. You can also make this recipe in advance and place it in a flask to consume throughout the day. Be careful though- caffeine is not an ideal ingredient in our alkaline journey, let's keep it as a treat, OK?
- ➢ During hot days, Argentineans like to have their yerba mate (*hierba mate*- in Spanish) with some apple juice. I like to add some lemon and grapefruit juice and ice cubes. Try it!

Cucumber Infused Lemon Ice Tea

Serves: 2-3

Ingredients:

- 2 cups cucumber
- 3 cups alkaline water
- 1 cup lemon juice
- Stevia to sweeten (optional)
- Ice cubes
- Mint leaves

Instructions:

- ➢ Boil one cup of water.
- ➢ Clean the cucumber thoroughly and remove the pith from both ends.
- ➢ Cut it into thin circles or little pieces.
- ➢ Place it in a bowl and add stevia.
- ➢ Pour the hot water on top and allow it to rest for 10 minutes.
- ➢ Meanwhile, mix the two cups of water and the lemon juice and place it in the fridge.
- ➢ Crush the ice in a coffee grinder or blender.
- ➢ Strain the cucumber water and add the ice cubes.

➤ Add in the cold lemon juice. Sprinkle some roughly chopped mint leaves on top and serve.

Red Bush (Rooibos) and Chili Tea

Serves: 4

Ingredients:

- 2 tablespoon Rooibos
- 5 tablespoons red chili flakes
- 4 cups alkaline water
- ½ cup lemon juice
- 2 tablespoon mint leaves
- Ice cubes

Instructions:

- ➤ Boil the water.
- ➤ Add in the Rooibos root.
- ➤ After 5 minutes, add in the chili flakes and switch off the heat.
- ➤ Allow it to stand for 5 minutes.
- ➤ Use a strainer to distil the water and place in a cup.
- ➤ Mix in the lemon juice and stir.
- ➤ Add in the ice cubes to make the liquid cold.
- ➤ Once it does, top it with the roughly chopped mint leaves and serve.
- ➤ You can sprinkle a little red chili flakes on top if you like it spicy.

Shave Grass Infused Tea

Serves: 2

Ingredients:

- 2 tablespoons shave grass (horsetail)
- 2 tablespoons red hibiscus flower
- 2 tablespoons mint leaves
- 2 tablespoons parsley leaves
- 2 cups alkaline water
- 1 teaspoon dates

Instructions:

- ➤ Clean the shave grass and hibiscus flowers thoroughly under running water.
- ➤ Boil the water.
- ➤ Remove a tablespoon full and pour over the dates to soften. Puree it in a blender.
- ➤ Add the shave grass and the hibiscus flowers to the water to allow it to release its flavor.
- ➤ Clean and roughly chop the mint and parsley leaves.
- ➤ Add in the mint and parsley leaves and switch off the heat.
- ➤ Allow it to stand for 10 minutes.

➢ Use a strainer to strain the liquid and serve with a teaspoon of date puree mixed in.

➢ Shave grass is great for a lot of things. It helps in reversing hair loss and promotes the growth of thick and shiny hair. It is also a great immunity builder! On a health side, helps burn fat and remove cellulite. I do recommend it a lot in my bestselling book: "Cellulite Killers".

Ginger Cumin Tea

Serves: 3-4

Ingredients:

- 1 ginger piece (about 2 inches)
- ¼ cup cumin seeds
- 4 cups alkaline water
- 2 tablespoons pepper
- 2 tablespoons parsley leaves
- Almond milk to taste

Instructions:

- ➢ Boil the water.
- ➢ Roughly chop the ginger and add it to the water.
- ➢ Add in ½ of the 1/4th cup of cumin to the boiling water and stir it. Boil for 5 minutes and turn off the heat.
- ➢ Place the rest of the seeds in a pan and allow it to roast on low heat.
- ➢ Strain the water and allow it to cool a bit before placing it in the fridge for 5 hours or overnight.
- ➢ You can serve it with ice cubes and add in some almond milk. Sprinkle some stevia, pepper, parsley leaves and toasted cumin on top.

Dandelion and Celery Tea

Serves: 5-6

Ingredients:

- 2 cups dandelion flowers
- 2 cups celery
- 6 cups alkaline water
- 1 tablespoon mint leaves
- 2 tablespoons cilantro leaves
- Stevia to sweeten

Instructions:

- ➢ Boil the water.
- ➢ Clean the dandelion flowers thoroughly by placing it under running water.
- ➢ Do the same with the celery.
- ➢ Add the celery and dandelion to the boiling water. Boil for 5 minutes
- ➢ Strain the water into a mug.
- ➢ Sweeten with stevia and add cilantro leaves on top. Serve hot.

Fennel Ice Tea

Serves: 5

Ingredients:

- 1 cup fennel seeds (plus 1 tablespoon)
- 5 cups alkaline water
- Ice cubes

Instructions:

- Boil the water.
- Add in the fennel seeds and allow it to boil for 30 minutes.
- Allow it to cool before placing it in the fridge for 6-12 hours.
- Pour it into a glass and top it with some fresh fennel seeds and ice cubes and serve.
- Enjoy!

CONCLUSION

Dear Reader,

Thanks again for taking interest in my book. I hope that you found some information and inspiration to start transforming your body and mind today.

All the recipes mentioned in this book were personally tested and I can vouch for their effectiveness in cleansing the body. I love these recipes as they are, but you can tweak them to suit your taste and preference. You could also experiment with the ingredients to come up with recipes of your own.

These tonics can be extremely effective if they are consumed regularly and can help you feel amazingly energized! So what are you waiting for? Hit that kitchen and start making these elixirs!

Remember to combine your alkaline drinks with a healthy and balanced diet of your choice. Whether you are Paleo, vegan, vegetarian, gluten-free, or just follow your own diet, your body will be happy if you feed it with more alkaline foods and drinks. <u>It will pay you back in vibrant health.</u>

The alkaline diet is not a diet. It is a lifestyle than can be combined with whatever diet you are following. It is my mission to show people how their lives can change if they "add more Alkalinity".

Here is another (basic) list of some alkaline and acidic foods for your reference.

Highly alkaline

Himalayan crystal salt, Cucumber, Green drinks, Grasses, Kale Kelp, Spinach, Broccoli, Parsley, Sprouts, Sea Vegetables (Kelp), Sprouted Beans and Sprouts

Moderately alkaline

Avocado, Basil, Beetroot, Bell Peppers, Capsicum, Celery, Endive, Tomato, Lettuce, Cabbage, Collard green, Spring Greens, Chives, Coriander, Garlic, Green Beans, Ginger, Mustard Greens, Onion, Red Onion Okra, Radish, Rocket or Arugula, Lemon and Lime, Soy Beans, Chia seeds, Quinoa, White Haricot Beans

Mildly alkaline

Asparagus, Artichokes, Brussels sprouts, Carrot, Cauliflower, Courgettes and Zucchini, Baby Potatoes, Leeks, Pumpkin, Pomegranate, Peas, Watercress, Swede Squash, Grapefruit,

Rhubarb, Coconut, Buckwheat, Tofu, Lentils, Goat milk, Almond milk, Herbs like Thyme and Mint, Spices like Ginger and Cumin, Olive Oil, Avocado Oil, Coconut Oil, Udo's Oil, Flax Oil etc

Apart from these, you can also make use of a few ingredients that are neutral to help add taste to your drinks. Those ingredients are as follows:

Cantaloupe, Watermelon, Sweet Cherry, Fresh Dates, Plum, Nectarine, Millet, Buckwheat, Rice milk, Soy Milk, Pecan Nuts, Brazil Nuts, Hazel Nuts, Grape Seed Oil and Sunflower Oil

Moderately Acidic

Butter, Mayonnaise, Natural Juice, Ketchup, Apricot, Apple, Banana, Blueberry Blackberry, Cranberry, Guava, Grapes, Mango, Peach, Orange, Pineapple, Papaya, Strawberry, Vegan Cheese, Goat's Cheese, Wheat Bread, Rye Bread, Whole meal bread, Whole meal Pasta, Wild Rice, Ocean Fish

Extremely Acidic

Tea, Coffee, Cocoa, Alcohol, Sweetened Fruit Juice, Honey, Jelly, Jam, Miso, Mustard, Soy Sauce, Rice Syrup Vinegar, Dried Fruit, Chicken, Beef, Eggs, Rice Syrup, Farmed Fish,

Shellfish, Pork Cheese, Artificial Sweeteners, Dairy and Mushroom

You will find a full list at:

http://bit.ly/AlkalineMarta

Your homework is to print it out and stick it on your fridge.

Which recipe was your favorite one? Please let me know in the review section on Amazon:

http://www.amazon.com/dp/B00TK386AY

For more inspiration and empowerment please visit:
www.holisticwellnessproject.com

Aside from the alkaline diet, wellness and recipes you will find plenty of articles on personal growth, happiness and motivation. I really hope that it can inspire you to take your life to a whole new level and create a new, balanced version of yourself. You will be surprised to see that Holistic Wellness Project is not just another health blog. I always say that health is not only about health. You must work on your body, mind and spirit in order to grow all areas of your life.

Finally, I invite you to join my interactive course: "The Alkaline Diet Lifestyle in 7 Simple Steps": www.AlkalineDietLifestyle.com

Not only will it teach you all you need to know about alkaline foods and diet, but it will also help you change your mindset when it comes to fitness and dieting in general. Motivation is really important, right?

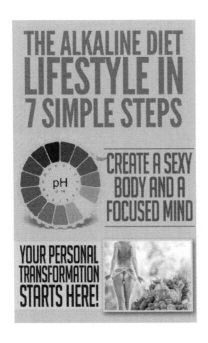

I hope to "see" you there.

I wish you lots of wellness and health. Body and mind transformation is an amazing journey of self-discovery!

CONNECT WITH ME:
http://www.facebook.com/HolisticWellnessProject

http://www.twitter.com/Marta_Wellness

https://www.linkedin.com/in/martatuchowska

http://www.goodreads.com/author/show/7520321.Marta_Tu
chowska

More Wellness Books by Marta Tuchowska:
www.amazon.com/author/mtuchowska

Printed in Great Britain
by Amazon.co.uk, Ltd.,
Marston Gate.